52 Weeks of Nutrition & Treats

A Nutritional Workbook
Ages 8 to Adult

S. Vella

To Vincent

∞

How to use this book:

Directions:

1. There will be 52 workbook pages with a nutrient or nutritional term for you to learn about, just as there are 52 weeks in a year.

2. You will need to complete the "Week" pages 1-52 in order, but may start any week of the year. Each page should only take about 5 to 15 minutes to complete!

3. Most weeks you will be learning about one particular nutrient and picking a "fresh food treat" that contains your week's nutrient. A "fresh food treat" is a non-processed food with preferably one ingredient, such as: fruits, veggies, beans, nuts, meat, etc. You will need to look up/research which foods contain your nutrient.

4. When picking out foods to try avoid anything that you may have allergies to or are not supposed to eat. Also, it is possible to consume too much of any one nutrient. You are solely responsible for any foods you try while completing this workbook.

5. Any time children need to look up/research information they will need a supervising adult's permission to use the internet.

When you see this:

*For my Body – Look up/research one or more interesting facts about your nutrient or termfor the week; something that it does for your body. For example: "It helps my eyesight, skin, brain, growth..." If applicable, answer a given question. Answers will vary.

*Investigate – Find out the definition and or meaning of your nutrient or term for the week. If applicable, answer a given question. Answers will vary.

*Artwork - This blank space is your own creative area. Younger children may wish to draw the food they've chosen or paste a picture from a magazine. Older children and adults may want to sketch something that either helps them remember what foods their nutrient is in or what it does for their body.

*Memorize – I think we all know what this means!

*Food Choice – Pick just one "fresh food treat" that is a good source of your week's nutrient that you would like to try. Purchase it during your regular weekly grocery store trip.

*Opinion – On a scale of 1 to 5, rate your food choice!
1=Awful,   2=Didn't care for it,   3=It was Okay,
4=Liked it,   5=Loved it!

For Group Use:

This book may be used by individuals or by classrooms, book clubs, home school groups, sports teams, men's groups, women's groups; you name it. It may be used by all sorts of groups, large and small, and by many different ages.

In a group setting you will need to know the amount of time you have to complete the workbook pages. Is your group meeting for an entire year or just a semester? You may have to do more than one page per week. Your group could choose which foods they would like to try and the group leader could bring those foods for everyone. Or you could rotate turns for individuals to bring their food selections.

These are just some suggestions for group use. Of course there are many different and creative ways you could do this!

Does this book cover <u>EVERYTHING</u> about nutrition?

    This book does not contain everything there is to know about nutrition. The purpose of this book is to cover, in a participatory way, many of the everyday nutrients that our human bodies need to thrive.

    The nutritional terms have been placed in logical order to make recollection of them easier. Each workbook page will not take long to complete. **By taking a few minutes to look something up, write a little, and sketch, you'll <u>retain knowledge</u> of your nutrient better than if you had just read a page about it. Compound this with thinking about your nutrient during your normal, weekly grocery store trip as you search for your "fresh food treat."**

    After completing this workbook you should have a good foundation in nutrition for the human body. You will have a broader understanding as to why different nutrients are important. You will have strengthened your ability to select good foods that you enjoy, while making healthier choices at the grocery store and elsewhere.

Table of Contents

Get Ready

Get Set

Begin

Week 1: Vitamins

Vitamins are essential in so many ways to the development and maintenance of the human body.

*Memorize:

Vitamin A
Vitamin C
Vitamin D
Vitamin E
Vitamin K
Vitamin B Complex

*Artwork: (Your artwork should be something that will help you remember what you are memorizing.)

Week 2: Vitamin A

*For My Body:

_____

_____

_____

_____

_____

*Artwork:

*Food Choice:	*Opinion:

Week 3: Vitamin C

*For My Body:

_____

_____

_____

_____

_____

*Artwork:

*Food Choice:	*Opinion:

Week 4: Vitamin D

*For My Body:

_____

_____

_____

_____

_____

*Artwork:

*Food Choice:	*Opinion:

Week 5: Vitamin E

*For My Body:

_____

_____

_____

_____

_____

*Artwork:

*Food Choice:	*Opinion:

Week 6: Vitamin K

*For My Body:

_____

_____

_____

_____

_____

*Artwork:

*Food Choice:	*Opinion:

Week 7: Vitamin B Complex

*Memorize:

Thiamine (B1)
Riboflavin (B2)
Niacin (B3)
Pantothenic Acid (B5)
B6
Biotin (B7)
Folate (B9)
B12

*Artwork: (Your artwork should be something that will help you remember what you are memorizing.)

Week 8: Thiamine (B1)

*For My Body:

_____

_____

_____

_____

_____

*Artwork:

*Food Choice:	*Opinion:

Week 9: Riboflavin (B2)

*For My Body:

_____

_____

_____

_____

_____

*Artwork:

*Food Choice:	*Opinion:

Week 10: Niacin (B3)

*For My Body:

_____

_____

_____

_____

_____

*Artwork:

*Food Choice:	*Opinion:

Week 11: Pantothenic Acid (B5)

*For My Body:

_____

_____

_____

_____

_____

*Artwork:

*Food Choice:	*Opinion:

Week 12: B6

*For My Body:

_____

_____

_____

_____

_____

*Artwork:

*Food Choice:	*Opinion:

Week 13: Biotin (B7)

*For My Body:

_____

_____

_____

_____

_____

*Artwork:

*Food Choice: *Opinion:

Week 14: Folate (B9)

*For My Body:

_____

_____

_____

_____

_____

*Artwork:

*Food Choice:	*Opinion:

Week 15: B12

*For My Body:

_____

_____

_____

_____

_____

*Artwork:

*Food Choice:	*Opinion:

Week 16: Minerals
Important nutrients that are needed by the body.

*Memorize:

Calcium
Magnesium
Phosphorus
Potassium
Sodium
Sulfur
(Electrolytes)

*Artwork: (Your artwork should be something that will help you remember what you are memorizing.)

Week 17: Calcium

*For My Body:

_____

_____

_____

_____

_____

*Artwork:

*Food Choice:	*Opinion:

Week 18: Magnesium

*For My Body:

_____

_____

_____

_____

_____

*Artwork:

*Food Choice:	*Opinion:

Week 19: Phosphorus

*For My Body:

_____

_____

_____

_____

_____

*Artwork:

*Food Choice:	*Opinion:

Week 20: Potassium

*For My Body:

_____

_____

_____

_____

_____

*Artwork:

*Food Choice:	*Opinion:

Week 21: Sodium

*For My Body: (The <u>good</u> things it does for you!)

_____

_____

_____

_____

*Investigate:
   Do fresh foods contain sodium?
   Does table salt contain sodium?

_____

_____

_____

_____

_____

_____

Week 22: Sulfur

*For My Body:

_____

_____

_____

_____

_____

*Artwork:

*Food Choice:	*Opinion:

Week 23: (Electrolytes)

*Investigate:

What is an electrolyte in nutrition?
What do electrolytes have to do with minerals?

_____

_____

_____

_____

_____

_____

*Artwork:

Week 24: Trace Minerals

Important nutrients that are used in very small amounts by the body.

*Memorize:

Iron
Copper
Fluoride
Iodine
Selenium
Zinc
Chromium
Manganese
Molybdenum
(Soil)

*Artwork: (Your artwork should be something that will help you remember what you are memorizing.)

Week 25: Iron

*For My Body:

_____

_____

_____

_____

_____

*Artwork:

*Food Choice:	*Opinion:

Week 26: Copper

*For My Body:

_____

_____

_____

_____

_____

*Artwork:

*Food Choice:	*Opinion:

Week 27: Fluoride

*Investigate:

　Why is fluoride sometimes added to drinking water?
　Why do some people believe fluoride to be harmful?

(Note: When you study nutrition there are bound to be disagreements between people on what is "healthy" or "natural." Fluoride is an excellent example of controversy in nutrition. The two questions posed above will address different sides of the fluoride debate without taking sides.)

_____

_____

_____

_____

_____

_____

*Artwork:

Week 28: Iodine

*For My Body:

_____

_____

_____

_____

_____

*Artwork:

*Food Choice: *Opinion:

Week 29: Selenium

*For My Body:

_____

_____

_____

_____

_____

*Artwork:

*Food Choice:	*Opinion:

Week 30: Zinc

*For My Body:

_____

_____

_____

_____

_____

*Artwork:

*Food Choice: ***Opinion:**

Week 31: Chromium

*For My Body:

_____

_____

_____

_____

_____

*Artwork:

*Food Choice:	*Opinion:

Week 32: Manganese

*For My Body:

_____

_____

_____

_____

_____

*Artwork:

*Food Choice:	*Opinion:

Week 33: Molybdenum

*For My Body:

_____

_____

_____

_____

_____

*Artwork:

*Food Choice:	*Opinion:

Week 34: (Soil)

*Investigate:

Are all soils the same?

Can soils contain minerals and or vitamins?

What, if any effect, does soil have on a crops mineral or vitamin content?

_____

_____

_____

_____

_____

_____

_____

*Artwork:

Week 35: Labels & Nutrition

*Investigate:

Step 1: Select three <u>packaged foods</u> from your cupboard, refrigerator, or freezer.

Step 2: Look for these terms on the packaging:
Fat, Cholesterol, Sodium, Carbohydrate, & Protein

Step 3: Compare the packaged foods. Are any of them unexpectedly high in sodium or fat? Carefully compare the five categories.

Step 4: Discuss your findings.

_____

_____

_____

_____

_____

_____

Week 36: Fats

*Investigate:

Why are fats often referred to as "good" and "bad" fats?
Which fat is generally going to be better for you, polyunsaturated or trans fat?

_____

_____

_____

_____

_____

_____

_____

*Artwork:

Week 37: Monounsaturated Fat & Polyunsaturated Fat

*For My Body:

_____

_____

_____

_____

_____

*Artwork:

*Food Choice:	*Opinion:

Week 38: Saturated Fat

*For My Body:

_____

_____

_____

_____

_____

*Artwork:

*Food Choice: *Opinion:

Week 39: Trans Fat
(Trans Fatty Acids)

*Investigate:

_____

_____

_____

_____

_____

_____

*Artwork:

Week 40: Cholesterol

*Investigate:
  What is cholesterol and how do you measure yours?

_____

_____

_____

_____

_____

_____

*Memorize:

HDL
LDL

Week 41: HDL
(high-density lipoprotein)

*Investigate:

_____

_____

_____

_____

_____

_____

*Artwork:

Week 42: LDL
(low-density lipoprotein)

*Investigate:

_____

_____

_____

_____

_____

_____

*Artwork:

Week 43: Protein

*For My Body:

_____

_____

_____

_____

*Investigate:
   What is a "complete protein"?

_____

_____

_____

_____

_____

*Food Choice:	*Opinion:

Week 44: Amino Acids

*Investigate:
   What is the difference between "Essential Amino Acids"
and "Non-Essential Amino Acids"?

_____

_____

_____

_____

_____

_____

*Artwork:

Week 45: Salt

We have already covered the mineral sodium. However, since sodium in the form of salt is often added to packaged foods it is important to study it.

*Investigate:
    What is Sodium-Chloride (or NaCl)?
    What could happen if you consumed too much salt?

_____

_____

_____

_____

_____

_____

_____

*Artwork:

Week 46: Carbohydrates

*Investigate:
   Are carbohydrates sugars? Why do we need them?

_____

_____

_____

_____

_____

_____

*Memorize:

Simple Carbs
Complex Carbs

Week 47: Simple Carbs

*Investigate:

What is the difference between a monosaccharide & a disaccharide?

What types of foods contain simple carbs?

_____

_____

_____

_____

_____

_____

*Artwork:

*Food Choice:	*Opinion:

Week 48: Complex Carbs

*Investigate:
   What is a polysaccharide?
   How do complex carbs fuel your body?
   What types of foods contain complex carbs?

_____

_____

_____

_____

_____

_____

*Memorize

Starch
Dietary Fiber

Week 49: Starch

*For My Body:

_____

_____

_____

_____

_____

*Artwork:

*Food Choice:	*Opinion:

Week 50: Dietary Fiber

*Investigate:

_____

_____

_____

_____

_____

_____

*Memorize:

Soluble Fiber
Insoluble Fiber

Week 51: Soluble Fiber

*For My Body:

_____

_____

_____

_____

_____

*Artwork:

*Food Choice:	*Opinion:

Week 52: Insoluble Fiber

* **For My Body:**

_____

_____

_____

_____

_____

* **Artwork:**

* **Food Choice:**	* **Opinion:**

COMPLETED!

Were any of the treats you picked out foods you tried for the first time? If so, which new things did you like?

After completing this nutritional workbook set one goal for yourself using the knowledge you've attained!

Keep this workbook as a journal that you can look back at any time you wish to review/remember something!

www.ingramcontent.com/pod-product-compliance
Lightning Source LLC
Chambersburg PA
CBHW081854280526
45789CB00007B/2696